INVESTING IN MEDICAL AND RECREATIONAL CANNABIS, BUY IN BEFORE, DURING AND AFTER LEGALIZATION

The DALIES. DE - 541-298-1085
Belgian TERVUREN
" MALINOIS

Mickey Dee

Table of Contents

INTRODUCTION

Marijuana also called weed, herb, pot, grass, bud, ganja, Mary Jane, and a vast number of other slang terms is a greenish gray mixture of the dried flowers of Cannabis sativa. Some people smoke marijuana in hand-rolled cigarettes called joints; in pipes, water pipes (sometimes called bongs), or in blunts (marijuana rolled in cigar wraps) Marijuana can also be used to brew tea and, particularly when it is sold or consumed for medicinal purposes, is frequently mixed into foods (edibles) such as brownies, cookies, or candies. Vaporizers are also increasingly used to consume marijuana. Stronger forms of marijuana include sinsemilla (from specially tended female plants) and concentrated resins containing high doses of marijuana's active ingredients, including honeylike hash oil, waxy budder, and hard amberlike shatter. These resins are increasingly popular among those who use them both recreationally and medically.

The main psychoactive (mind-altering) chemical in marijuana, responsible for most of the intoxicating effects that people seek, is delta-9-tetrahydrocannabinol (THC). The chemical is found in resin produced by the leaves and buds primarily of the female cannabis plant. The plant also contains more than 500 other chemicals, including more than 100 compounds that are chemically related to THC, called cannabinoids.

Introduction to Cannabis Stocks and Investments

Legalization is spreading and continues to make a strong case for informed cannabis investment. In recent months, we've witnessed a sea of change in the position of cannabis in the U.S. marketplace, coupled with burgeoning investment opportunities. To date, nine states permit recreational marijuana. The District of Columbia, approves. And most states have legalized medicinal pot use.

Major breakthroughs have continued this year. In early 2018, California became the latest to legalize recreational use.

Most recently, Vermont became the first state to legalize marijuana not by a ballot measure, but by formal enactment of a law through its legislature.

There is no time like the present to invest in cannabis, and the satellite industries supporting its production. Here are some factors that may influence your stock selections and earning potential, should you decide to invest in this emerging sector.

Growers and dispensaries now expect legislation to prevent the federal government from interfering with states' legalization, and that's good news for marijuana stocks. Although an actual federal law that declares cannabis legal might not occur for years, state regulation is proving to be up to the task of regulating the substance.

Because state law controls cannabis sales, the sector is working with something of a patchwork. Even amid this complexity, there is financial opportunity. Companies that offer compliance tools for the industry are on the rise.

Growers are now looking forward to the day, likely not far off on the horizon, when banks may freely provide services to the sector. Should the federal government ease restrictions as it is expected to do, watch for U.S. marijuana stocks to skyrocket. At that point it will also be easier for international suppliers to enter the U.S. landscape.

Types of Cannabis Companies

A wide variety of businesses make up and support the cannabis sector and are well positioned for financial growth.

There are the growers themselves. These are known as "plant touching" companies, such as California's Terra Tech corporation.

Then there are the companies that supply energy to the growers. They are in high demand by the large-scale indoor operations that would put too much pressure on the grid if they didn't have alternative solutions.

A variety of other technology companies are gearing up for the growth of this industry, as are companies that provide a spectrum of supplies.

There's also Canna-Hub, a developer and manager of cannabis real estate, also known as cannabis communities. Canna-Hub of California has two such developments — and both have transformed small-town economies.

Another ancillary business type helps with employee management. A company called Wurk is an early entrant in the field. Wurk helps cannabis-related firms handle tax rules, payroll deposits, and regulation. With operations in 27 states, Wurk can connect businesses to banks that will work with legal marijuana companies.

Compliance software shows a great deal of promise in this area as well. A vital need in the cannabis sector is the automation of reporting to government agencies. A state that makes cannabis legal has to follow through with regulation. The state will track every action taken with every plant, from seed to retail. Technology is relieving business owners of many small administrative tasks that would otherwise add up to a full-time job.

A leader in this market segment is Green Bits. It's a firm that provides dispensaries with everything they need to stay in compliance with state rules and regulations. Compliance software is so vital that Green Bits now serves some 1,000 dispensaries in 12 states

Tiger Global, a New York venture capital firm and an early investor in many major tech powerhouses including LinkedIn and Facebook, has now invested in Green Bits. Casa Verde Capital, owned by Snoop Dogg, has also invested in Green Bits, helping to bring the software company more than $19 million in funding.

Kush Bottles

Analysts expect this packaging maker's impressive revenue growth, spurred by California's legalization of medical and recreational cannabis, to rise significantly in the years ahead. California requires child-proof packaging for pot — one of Kush's strong suits.

AbbVie Inc.

The maker of the FDA-approved cannabis-based drug Marinol, a digestive aid for chemotherapy patients and AIDS sufferers, focuses on U.S. markets. This is a powerful, established front-runner. Yet most analysts believe the best strategy with any stocks is diversification, rather than going solely with a stock such as AbbVie, or relying only on the U.S. market.

Aurora Cannabis.

Another licensed producer of medical marijuana in Canada, Aurora Cannabis, Inc., is currently the fastest growing North American cannabis company. With this company, you'll want to keep an eye on potential dilution of stock.

Canopy Growth Corp.

Medical marijuana company and the Yukon Liquor Corporation entered into an agreement. Canopy will supply Yukon with cannabis products in light of Canada's forthcoming nationwide legal market for recreational cannabis. This represents a collaboration with the government of Yukon. Canopy is also a selected retail partner in Manitoba, Newfoundland and Labrador.

How to Start Investing

New cannabis stock investors have a spectrum of entry points available. Which one is right for you? The one that suits your current investment style is likely best.

There are plenty of opportunities in this space to purchase stocks over the counter. Note that this method takes a good eye for inspecting balance sheets. It also means achieving a familiarity with financial facts, such as the companies' asset-to liability ratios, and likelihood of stock dilution. So before jumping in, put the search engines to use and read.

HOW TO INVEST IN MARIJUANA STOCKS

Before moving on, it's important to note that investing in cannabis is not limited to growers or retailers. There are numerous companies providing ancillary services to the industry, as well as many derivative plays, like pharma and biotech companies making cannabinoid-based drugs and service/product providers that used to operate outside the marijuana industry but have gotten on board since legalization.

The over-the-counter issue

While multiple states in the U.S. have legalized

cannabis for either recreational or medical uses, allowing companies to thrive, the plant is still illegal on a Federal level – classified as a Schedule I drug by the DEA. This has made it difficult for many companies to get listed on the Nasdaq or the NYSE.

Seeking alternative avenues to raise capital, some businesses have gone public by trading on over-the-counter exchanges. This means that many publicly traded cannabis companies are not subject to the same level of scrutiny that major exchanges and the SEC impose.

"The over-the-counter exchanges present challenges. They're not taken as seriously as the bigger exchanges, and they also allow for a greater degree of latitude in terms of the quality of the company that will trade on them. As a result, many of the companies that have something to do with cannabis probably shouldn't be there. They got there because entrepreneurs thought it was the only way they could get access to capital; there was somebody that had a publicly traded vehicle that seemed like it would be a good fit," Leslie Bocskor, investment banker and President of cannabis advisory firm Electrum Partners.

Having said this, he added that not all OTC or penny stocks are to be avoided at all costs. "There is a prejudice against low priced stocks that I think we need to get away from as an industry and start looking towards reverse splitting our stocks, having fewer numbers of shares and higher prices because the optics on it are better," Bocskor voiced.

How to hash out the bad weed stocks

So, we're still faced with the same question as we were a few paragraphs ago: how does one pick good cannabis stocks and avoid bad ones?

While it is always recommended that retail investors do their own due diligence, going over hundreds of filings and corporate documents can be hard and time-consuming. Moreover, most people usually don't have access to the resources needed to make an informed assessment of a company.

But there are options. One of them is investing in ETFs like the ones mentioned above: Horizons Marijuana Life Sciences Index ETF and the ETFMG Alternative Harvest ETF. These instruments make it easy to invest in cannabis stocks that have already been pre-selected by teams of analysts who've conducted the necessary due diligence and decided to include certain companies in these ETFs.

Another option for those looking to build out their own portfolios is recurring to investment advisors and stock pickers like Alan Brochstein or Jeff Siegel of Green Chip Stocks.

"A lot of the Canadian cannabis stocks are quite overvalued right now," Siegel warns.We are telling the readers to start focusing on some US cannabis stocks, as this is the next big market. Companies like MariMed (OTC: MRMD) and Innovative Industrial Properties (NYSE: IIPR) are doing quite well as the US cannabis market becomes more attractive."

The six steps to retail investing

So, to make things simpler, here's a list of six steps you should be taking when investing in cannabis stocks – or any other sort of security, for that matter.

Step 1: Research the company

Always start by researching the company or companies you'll be investing in. Check SEC filings and other documents required by diverse regulatory agencies. Also, read the latest news on these companies in site likes Yahoo Finance and get a feel for the market sentiment using Twitter or Stocktwits.

Step 2: Determine the amount to invest

As a rule of thumb, never invest more than you can afford to lose. While good research will often lead to strong returns, this will not necessarily be the case. Stocks are volatile and contingencies sometimes unpredictable.

In relation to this point, Brochstein says, "I find many people place too much confidence in just one or two ideas. In a start-up industry, which is what legal cannabis is in many ways, it's not easy to pick the winners. If you go back to the late 1990s, a lot of the companies that many expected to be winners didn't even survive three years. My longer-term focused model portfolios typically have a dozen names in them."

Step 3: Decide on your timeline

Deciding on when to buy and when to sell is crucial. Try and figure out what your thresholds are beforehand. So, for instance, establish a rule:

"if the stock falls below X or surges above Y, I'll sell."

Step 4: Pick a broker

Recommended Broker

Ally Invest has phenomenal research reports which help navigate and inform you of marijuana stocks that have potential. On top of that, they have some of the industries lowest fees for stock trading. Depending on how much you fund your account with you can get some cash bonuses and trade commission free.

Once you've gone through the initial steps, you'll be ready to actually buy your shares. You can go old-school, with a brick and mortar broker like Scottrade or sign up for an online broker such as E*Trade or Interactive Brokers. Both options will allow you to buy and sell stocks once you've registered and funded your account.

Step 5: Buy the stock

This step may sound self-explanatory, but it's a bit more complex than it seems.

"There are generally two types of 'buy' orders: market order and a limit order. A market order will execute the purchase at the present market price, while a limit order will only execute if the price falls at or below the limit price. Although a limit price might give an investor a lower price of entry, there is no guarantee that the limit order will execute," Benzinga's Thomas Rudy explains.

Step 6: Sell the stock

Once you feel you've generated enough returns from a stock, it'll be time to sell. Again, you can sell the stock with a market order or a limit order. Use your proceeds to reinvest or just spend them. Life is meant for living!

Trading around a core

One of the processes that have helped Brochstein

perform well in his model portfolios has been what he likes to call "trading around a core."

This strategy takes advantage of the inherent volatility in these stocks, The way it works is that you sell incrementally when the stocks are rallying or buy incrementally when the stocks are declining," he explains.

"It's important to make sure that the position deserves to be a holding, but if you are confident in the long-term prospects for the stock, varying your exposure can allow you to 'buy the dip' or 'sell the rip' and not get left on the sidelines or get buried if the stock moves higher after you trim your position or lower after you add to it. To be real clear, if you go 'all in' on a stock and make it 50% of your portfolio, what are you going to do if it drops further? If you sell out of what you think is a great long-term holding because it has reached a level you didn't expect, will you then be willing to pay more to buy it back in the future if it never falls.

MARIJUANA ADVANCES OF THE 21ST CENTURY

Cannabinoids are the main chemicals in marijuana. In recent years, various research and experiments have resulted in production of high CBD marijuana strains and in a large percent of these strains, THC is non-existent. But it doesn't take research to know that inhaling any kind of smoke into your lungs is bad for your health. Because of this, new ways to administer medical marijuana are being invented so the patient no longer has to smoke to medicate. Cannabinoids can be so beneficial; the human brain has two built-in cannabinoid receptors, which regulate certain body functions. These are just some of the advances in the research and study of high CBD medical marijuana in the 21st century.

Cannabinoids are the main medicinal ingredient in marijuana. While THC is the main psychoactive ingredient, cannabinoids are known to have anti-psychotic properties, which counter the effects of THC. With this in mind, production labs are now growing strains of marijuana that contain a high concentration of CBD's. Some of these strains have CBD concentrations as high as 20%, which allow people living with illness to benefit from medical marijuana without the high associated with THC. Up until recently, a big concern for some, was the fact that in order to use medical marijuana, an individual had to get high as a side effect. That made many question the intentions of a so-called medical marijuana patient. Does he or she really have an ailment or do they just want to get high? With high CBD strains, getting high is no longer a factor while medicating with marijuana. Therefore these strains will make it safe for everyone, from small kids to elderly adults, to medicate without concern of any intoxicating effects. The development of high CBD marijuana should continue to help completely remove the stigma from its medical use.

There was a time when if a patient wanted to use medical marijuana, not only did they have to get high, they had to smoke it. Smoking anything involves inhaling harmful chemicals into your lungs that were released as the medium burned. Today there are numerous ways of administering and self-dosing medical marijuana. They range from vaporizing, cooking, and drinks, to oral sprays and tinctures. Vaporizing involves heating marijuana to a point where it produces a vapor, then inhaling the vapor into the lungs. For smokers, vaporizing is the non-smoked method most often recommended as an alternative to smoking because vaporization releases about 5 compounds, whereas smoking marijuana releases about 111 different compounds. Cooking with medical marijuana involves heating marijuana and butter. The butter traps the chemicals and is then used in any dish of the patient's choice. Various drinks can also be made with the butter or some can be bought already made. Tonics and tinctures are made when marijuana is soaked in an alcohol solution, transferring the cannabinoids to the liquid. The tincture can then be rubbed on skin, taken by drops or sprayed into the mouth and put into foods and drink recipes as well. Medical marijuana also comes in the forms of ready-made candy and various other sweets, all of the high CBD form. Still, as with any type of medication, the attractively packaged items should be kept out of reach of children.

Cannabinoids in medical marijuana have the same effect as the cannabinoids that already occur in every person. The human body naturally produces cannabinoids similar to those of marijuana on its own. Researchers at Brown University have shown that the brain produces anandamide, which is a pain suppressing cannabinoid. This naturally produced chemical affects the CB1 and CB2 cannabinoid receptors of the human nervous and immune systems respectively. These cannabinoids regulate physiological processes including appetite, pain-sensation, mood, and memory. They also regulate sleep patterns and act as natural inflammatory agents. CBD's from medicinal marijuana have been recognized for their ability to act as antioxidants in the brain. Researchers have found that cannabinoids are capable of not only cleansing damaged brain cells, but also triggering the production of new brain cells. This has led to high CBD marijuana being researched as a treatment for concussions in professional athletes. With the added CBD's from medicinal marijuana, patients can be treated for a variety of other ailments and conditions. The marijuana could be prescribed for anything from simple appetite loss to pain caused multiple sclerosis; because a lot of times, the ones produced by the body are not enough.

Since the days of Reefer Madness, the study and research along with negative views of marijuana have come a long way. Science is giving us a clearer understanding of what is in it and how we can utilize those ingredients to benefit and treat ailments of the afflicted. Medical marijuana no longer has to be smoked. More importantly, high CBD marijuana will not get a patient high, at all. The fact that the human body makes and uses its own cannabinoids anyway, should be an eye opener to the medical field. Marijuana as a medicine is as or more effective than almost any prescribed drug on earth and research is proving that it is so much safer. With the high from THC being negated in high CBD marijuana, and new ways of medicating without smoking; there is no longer a reason for selfish organizations to keep something with the potential to be so beneficial, from those who would clearly benefit from it.

INVESTING IN THE CANNABIS INDUSTRY

Emerging sectors like the cannabis industry have often attracted investors hoping to be among the first to capitalize on the potential growth and high returns of what they believe are untapped markets or products that may be popular in the future.

While it's true that some new sectors have been successful for some investors, such as those who invested early in internet-based companies, the chase for the next big investment can lead investors to speculate on trends and bet on industries and products with no proven record or history of success.

The cannabis industry in particular has grown quickly in recent years as a number of jurisdictions, including Canada and certain U.S. states, have explored new laws around the sale and use of cannabis. In Canada, this initially began with the legalization of cannabis for medicinal purposes, which prompted a number of companies to express interest in entering the market and approaching investors who were keen to get in on what they believed was the next big thing.

Cannabis regulation in Canada may continue to evolve over time as the federal government plans to legalize its recreational use. Because of this, many cannabis companies are promising investors the opportunity to capitalize on the potential for considerable future growth. A number of companies are looking to expand into the U.S. where some states have authorized sale and use of cannabis for medicinal or recreational purposes, even though it remains prohibited at the federal level.

Investing in a cannabis company comes with a number of risks that could negatively affect an investment at any time. There remains a large amount of uncertainty in this emerging sector, especially as laws and business models continue to evolve.

Some investors may see others flocking toward an emerging sector and can be compelled to follow out of fear of missing out on an opportunity. However, behavioural insights into the way that people make decisions about money has shown that investors who follow other investors' behaviour are more likely to invest in speculative bubbles that could burst. If that happens, investors could stand to lose some or all of their investment.

Businesses in the cannabis industry

The rapid expansion of the cannabis industry has created opportunities for a number of new companies to develop products, technologies and services beyond just the cultivation and distribution of cannabis itself. There are now a number of businesses operating under the umbrella of the cannabis industry, even if their business does not actually grow or sell cannabis products directly, making it possible to invest in a cannabis company without investing in the cultivation or distribution of cannabis itself.

Some examples of businesses operating within the cannabis industry include:

Agriculture technology: Businesses that support the innovation and development of equipment required to cultivate cannabis, such as automated fertilizer systems, greenhouse technologies and improved lighting systems.

Ancillary products and services: Businesses that offer products that complement the cannabis industry as a whole, which can include products like a cannabis breathalyzer to laboratories that test cannabis products. This also includes companies that provide insurance to cultivators as well as those that create consumer packaging for products.

Biotechnology: Businesses that focus on the pharmaceutical applications of cannabis by developing treatments to target illnesses and diseases.

Consulting services: Businesses that respond to the complexity of rules and regulations around cannabis between different jurisdictions. They may provide services to assist with licensing, zoning or advising on operational processes.

Consumption devices: Businesses that create products that people use to consume cannabis.

Cultivation and retail: Businesses that grow and sell cannabis, and are often the types of businesses that most people think of when discussing the cannabis industry.

Cannabis products and extracts: Businesses that sell cannabidiol products, edibles, topicals, drinks and other products.

Holding companies: Businesses that typically own a considerable number of voting shares in a variety of cannabis companies, allowing them to influence the management and affairs of the companies held.

Industrial hemp: Businesses that provide products using industrial hemp, which is different than cannabis and may have numerous applications and uses, including creating consumer products like paper and clothing, as well as building materials, fuel and foods.

Organic farms: Businesses that provide organically-grown cannabis to other companies or sell to consumers directly, relying on the increasing demand for organic products and services to drive the business's growth.

Investing risks

All investments come with some amount of risk. Generally, the higher the potential return of an investment, the higher the risk. There is no guarantee that you will actually get a higher return by accepting more risk. Learn more about the risk-return relationship.

When you invest in the cannabis industry, you're exposed to different types of risk that can affect your potential return. Some common risks include:

No guarantee of success

Despite the rapid growth of companies in the cannabis sector, there remains no guarantee that their businesses are profitable or will be in the future. Many cannabis companies are hedging their success on the future distribution and sale of their product, despite the fact that many rules and regulations around distribution and sale are still in the process of being established.

Some early medical cannabis companies were not successful, with some often failing to provide investors with adequate disclosure about the barriers to entering the industry (such as licenses required to grow cannabis) and other work needed to create a profitable business. While these disclosure requirements have been addressed by Canadian securities regulators, the risks of investing in this emerging industry still remain. As with any investment, there is no guarantee that an investment in the cannabis industry will provide any return or income.

Government regulation

The governments and regulators in many of the

jurisdictions that are exploring new cannabis laws have yet to fully establish the framework for how and where cannabis products can be sold. For example, there may be some restrictions on the stores that are permitted to sell cannabis, as well as rules about branding and advertising that could affect a consumer's ability to find and purchase products. These sorts of challenges can affect a company's ability to sell its products and make a profit, which in turn could reduce the value of your investment in the company.

As regulation continues to evolve and the cannabis industry grows, new companies will enter the industry and compete with existing cannabis businesses. Increased competition may compel a company you have invested in to adjust its business model, adjust the prices of its products, or make other changes in order to stay competitive. This may affect the value of your investment.

Legal considerations

Cannabis companies must abide by all the laws and regulations of the jurisdictions in which they operate, which can vary from country to country. Should laws change, the company may be required to adjust its operations to comply with the law or risk having legal action taken against it. In some cases, this may mean ending its business.

In the U.S., some states have authorized the sale and use of cannabis, but it still remains illegal under federal law. Authorities in the U.S. could choose to enforce federal law at any time, putting any company with cannabis-related activities in any U.S. state at risk of being prosecuted and having its assets seized.

Investing in a company that does business in a place where the law either prohibits cannabis or is unclear about its use puts your money at risk. If legal action is taken against a company in which you have invested, you could stand to lose your entire investment.

While laws and regulations around the sale and use of cannabis in Canada are changing, there are still a number of rules in place to guide the way that cannabis companies operate. If a business does not comply with these rules, it could have legal action taken against it and you could stand to lose your investment.

Pricing and taxation

Government-mandated pricing and taxation on cannabis products may also pose a risk to the success of a cannabis company. Cannabis products, especially those intended for recreational use, should be priced below their black market value in order to attract consumers. If the government prices cannabis products too high, or if black market dealers undercut prices of products available in stores, the companies growing and selling the products may not be able to sell enough product to make a profit.

Inflated share prices

Opportunities to invest in new cannabis companies or existing companies expanding their business into the cannabis industry have generated a high level of interest among investors looking to get in on a new trend with the expectation of quick growth. However, these investments can be highly speculative, and the cost of an investment in a cannabis company may be based on the expectation of its future success rather than its current performance.

In some cases, companies that have simply announced their intent to develop a cannabis business have seen an immediate rise in their stock price, before there is even a viable business in place. Investors who buy shares in these companies risk paying an inflated price for an investment that may never increase in value.

Dilution

As the popularity for cannabis-related products grows, companies have to scale up their operations to meet the demand, which may include building larger facilities, buying additional equipment and hiring additional employees. This can cost considerable amounts of money, and if a company doesn't have the funds required to expand its operations, it may choose to raise money by issuing additional shares.

When companies issue additional shares to raise money, it comes at the expense of existing shareholders, whose percentage ownership decreases proportionally to the number of new shares created. This is known as dilution. If you hold shares in a company that continuously raises money by issuing more shares, your investment will decrease in value.

High operating costs

The costs associated with developing and

operating a commercial cannabis company can be considerable. Growing and selling cannabis requires specialized and large-scale agriculture facilities and enormous amounts of power and capital in order to operate. Construction and energy costs can greatly increase a company's overhead, and as companies scale up in order to meet demand, the costs of constructing new buildings may undercut profitability, especially if there are significant cost overruns or construction delays that impact a company's ability to produce and deliver its product.

As an investor, you should understand the company's business plan and how it intends to earn a profit, as well as the related risks, costs of doing business and time it may take for the business to become profitable. There is no guarantee that a company will be successful in generating profits or increasing its stock value.

Getting information before you invest

If you are considering investing in a cannabis company, you should first take some steps toward researching the investment opportunity and considering how the investment will help meet your financial goals:

Review disclosure documents. Companies offering investors the opportunity to invest

are required to provide specific disclosure documents, such as a prospectus listing statement or an offering memorandum, which contains information about the business, its management, operations and business risks, including the nature of its operations in specific countries and states, as well as how it complies with laws in each jurisdiction in which it conducts business.

Read official materials. Annual reports, management's discussion and analysis, news releases and other official company materials can provide information about whether the company is making or losing money, information about its financial statements

and comments from management on how the company has performed, as well as any industry trends or events that may have affected the company's operations.

Speak with an advisor. Advisors can answer questions about particular investment products and assist you with selecting investments that can help you achieve your financial goals.

CANNABIS INVESTMENT: CANADIAN CANNABIS STOCKS

Canadian cannabis stocks have been on investors' lips the last year. When it comes to cannabis investment, there are so many large and small companies on different exchanges, market watchers are left wondering what Canadian cannabis stocks are out there to choose from? Plus, what are the legal implications and what are the risks in this sector? The Canadian cannabis sector is taking huge steps in establishing guidelines for their product and finding international opportunities in the medical landscape.

Business in cannabis has expanded into massive levels of investment thanks to opportunities in various stock listings. In Canada, cannabis companies can seek public investment through stock listings on the Toronto Stock Exchange (TSX), its smaller sibling market TSX Venture (TSXV) and the Canadian Securities Exchange (CSE).

For those interested in cannabis investment, here's a look at a variety of publicly traded Canadian cannabis stocks. The list includes cannabis and hemp focused stocks divided by the respective Canadian exchange.

Cannabis Investment: Stocks on the TSX

The TSX has seen leaders of the cannabis industry join its listing and offer investors a new venue into cannabis ventures. These include massive license producers (LPs) expanding their product and brands overseas.

Aphria (TSX:APH)

Also licensed under the ACMPR, much like other companies on the Canadian cannabis stocks, Aphria is located in Leamington, Ontario. The company self-describes itself as "truly powered by sunlight", which they state allows for natural growing conditions to produce safe medical cannabis products.

Aphria made its strategic entrance to the US cannabis market through Liberty Health Sciences (CSE:LHS; OTCBB:LHSIF), which seeks and partners with cannabis companies in the US. Its first market is in Florida. Despite its interest in the American market, the company was forced to dump its assets south of the border due to regulations issues with the TMX Group. Aphria sold its cannabis investment in an Arizona producer to Liberty Health and plans to let go of its own stake in Liberty Health.

Aurora Cannabis (TSX:ACB)

List for cannabis investment is Aurora Cannabis. This company is currently fast at work on the development of their Aurora Sky facility, an 800,000 square foot hybrid greenhouse, which obtained its cultivation license from Health Canada, the country's regulator.

As part of their most recent quarterly update to shareholders the company revealed it had reached $11.7 million in revenue for the second quarter of their fiscal 2018 year. The company also shared some details on one of their most recent partnerships, an investment deal with Liquor Stores N.A. meant to plan for the creation of cannabis retail outlets.

The company explained its new investee will convert existing retail locations into specific cannabis outlets while also looking for new spaces to develop.

The company completed its full acquisition of CanniMed Therapeutics and managed the delisting of the company as it became an asset for Aurora.

Now the company continues its path of cannabis investments and acquisitions by announcing a deal to purchase MedReleaf (TSX:LEAF). The deal is worth over C$3 billion to buy all the issued and outstanding common shares of MedReleaf.

Graduating to the TSX reflects the amazing progress we have made since listing on the CSE in August last year and represents yet another important milestone for CannTrust as we continue our successful journey as one of Canada.

This year the Canadian cannabis stock managed to complete a $15,000,000 mortgage financing deal for its greenhouse facility in Niagara.

Canopy Growth (TSX:WEED)

Most investors in the cannabis investment space

will know of Canopy Growth, the largest Canadian cannabis stock, having been the first cannabis organization to surpass the $1 billion market cap.

Canopy holds producers Tweed and Bedrocan under its umbrella. Tweed's production facility is located in the old Hershey factory in Smith Falls, Ontario, while its breeding facility was completed. The company believes the state-of-the-art facility is the first of its kind and will form the foundation of new Canadian-bred genetics.

Canopy regularly announces new deals and partnerships with international emerging markets. Late in 2017, the company announced a deal that sent a signal to the entire industry. Constellation Brands (NYSE:STZ), a massive alcohol producer in the US, invested in 9.9 percent equity of Canopy, which signaled the increased credibility of the cannabis business to the overall market.

Following in the steps of Cronos Group (NASDAQ:CRON), Canopy announced its intentions to list on the New York Stock Exchange. The company is trading in the US under the ticker symbol "CGC", giving Americans interested in cannabis investment another stock to choose from.

Cronos Group (TSX:CRON)

Next on stock list for cannabis investment is Cronos, a Canadian licensed producer with assets in international markets such as Australia and Israel. This year the company became the first Canadian LP to list its common shares on the Nasdaq Global Markets. The company does not own any assets in the US but has indicated it wishes to enter the market once all legal issues are cleared for the drug.

Since the start of the year, the company has been raising money with a couple of different bought deals, worth C$46 million and C$100 million separately. The company upgraded its Canadian shares to the TSX on May 22.

MedReleaf is one of the Canadian cannabis stocks whose company is working to advance the knowledge available on the therapeutic benefits of cannabis for patient care. At the Canaccord cannabis investor day conference, they revealed throughout their four primary areas of focus included the Canadian medical cannabis market and opportunities over in the international market.

The company was rumored to begin a process of making players know the company was available for the taking. The rumors were then confirmed once an acquisition deal with Aurora Cannabis was announced.

THE GREEN ORGANIC

Publicly launched this year, this company counts with the backing from major Canadian LP Aurora Cannabis, even appointing Cam Battley, chief corporate officer with Aurora, into TGOD's board of directors.

The company was able to close its initial public offering with gross proceeds worth $132,263,225 under the IPO thanks in part to issue an additional 36,236,500 units of the company, and including the over-allotment units to financial institutions.

Cannabis Investment: Stocks on the TSXV

Previously known as the Canadian Venture

Exchange, the TSX Venture Exchange is the sibling listing from the larger Toronto Stock Exchange. This listing offers a variety of Canadian cannabis stocks ranging from growers to biotech companies looking for cannabinoid (CBD) therapies.

Vivo Cannabis Inc (VVCIF) (.66)

ABcann Global (TSXV:ABCN)

First on TSXV stock list for cannabis investment is ABcann became public this year with a complete TSXV listing. This licensed producer is set to expand with additions to their staff and new 100,000-square-foot facility set to add to their current 625 kilograms per year production.

The Canadian cannabis stock evaluates its product under a climate-controlled chamber, which allows it to put out a uniform product and be safer when it comes to new Health Canada randomized inspections on cannabis from its producers. In July, ABcann announced its listing on the OTCQB Marketplace and Frankfurt Stock Exchange. Prior to that, it–together with Cannabis Wheaton–

announced the signing of an agreement for the first tranche of a $15 million placement.

Auxly Cannabis Group (TSXV:XLY)

(CBWTF) (.66)

Previously known as Cannabis Wheaton Income, this cannabis investment company operates employing the streaming business plan made popular in the mining sector. Therefore Auxly scans the sector and provides funding support for other companies in the investment space. In return, the company gets minority equity interests and a percentage of the cultivation.

President Hugo Alves told INN the cannabis investment company overcame an unsuccessful offering deal with two financial banking institutions to continue their financing business with other cannabis businesses in Canada.

BLOCKSTRAIN TECHNOLOGY

BLOCKStrain is a software company working on a blockchain-based platform for supply chains management in the cannabis industry. The company has signed deals with cannabis producers WeedMD (TSXV:WMD) and Abattis Bioceuticals (CSE:ATT) for the use of its platform.

Delta 9 Cannabis (VRNDF) (1.26)

Next on our stock list for cannabis investment is Delta 9. The company is a cannabis producer located in Manitoba and currently in the running for one of the four master licenses set to be awarded to companies for the involvement of the upcoming cannabis market in that province. They partnered with Canopy Growth (TSX:WEED) for their business development under their CraftGrow program.

"We are already working closely on a project to jointly serve the growing market in Manitoba; this project brings Delta 9's craft grown cannabis products to a wider national audience through Canopy Growth's well-established CraftGrow network," Delta 9 CEO John Arbuthnot said.

Emblem 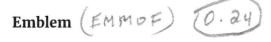 *(EMMOF)* *(0.24)*

Like most other Canadian cannabis investment stocks, Emblem is a licensed producer in Canada, currently using the latest in indoor grow science. The company's new facility located in Ontario was designed with a purpose to cultivate and cure cannabis for medicinal use. Emblem gave the go-ahead in December 2016 from Health Canada to begin production of cannabis oil.

Emerald Health Botanicals 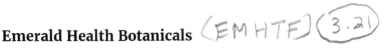 (EMHTF) (3.21)

Emerald Health Botanicals, previously Emerald Health therapeutics, is a licensed medical marijuana producer under MMPR. As a federal research grant recipient, the Canadian cannabis stock conducts research and development into the characterization of cannabis strains and cultivation technologies. It also collaborates with academic and medical research to help gain further understanding of the effect of cannabis on humans.

FluroTech (FLURF) (0.33)

For those wanting to gain exposure to cannabis investment without directly investing in an LP, technology is a good option. FluroTech is a technology company working on a cost-effective testing platform for the cannabis industry at large. The company's proprietary CompleTest employing fluorescence spectroscopy technology to measure specific contents of the product.

The company began trading publicly on the TSXV on June 12 after obtaining approval from the exchange. "It is expected the company will launch its marketing program to licensed producers with direct sales of the portable and desktop testing devices for heavy metal and potency tests this summer," FluroTech said.

HARVEST ONE CANNABIS

(HRVOF) 0.69

Harvest One conducts its business thanks to three different units, United Greeneries provides the horticultural arm while Satipharm AG serves the medical arm. Those two are under the Harvest One umbrella. Each business is strategically located with supportive regulatory frameworks in place. United Greeneries has received a Canadian medicinal cannabis cultivation license. The company announced on May 9 it had completed its first international shipment, with product heading to Australia.

HEXO CORP

The Hydropothecary Corporation (HEXO) 6.77

Also a licensed producer, this cannabis investment

option sells their product through their website and grows it under a glass roof greenhouse, which makes it so their crops receive direct sunlight.

Hydropothecary went public in March following a couple of false starts, according to the Financial Post, the company joined the TSXV due to the potential for legalization on the recreational market.

This year the company announced the appointment of Dr. Terry Lake, former B.C. Minister of Health, as their new vice-president of corporate social responsibility.

ICC Labs   *(ICC.VN) (1.620)*

This licensed integrated Canadian cannabis stock operates out of Uruguay, a leader in the legal cannabis investment space and a model many other countries have looked for a similar strategy. ICC is also investing in cannabis research to improve understanding of its physical uses and medical benefits.

The Canadian cannabis stock obtained two licenses to enter the medical cannabis market in Colombia, adding to its reach in the Latin American cannabis investment market.

INDIVA LTD (NDVAF) 0.47

INDIVA is a relatively new player in the cannabis investment space, their focus is on the supply of medical cannabis. Through an acquisition, this company holds a licensed producer with an indoor cannabis facility in Ontario.

The Canadian cannabis stock signed an exclusive agreement with Medropharm GmbH and Greenfields Health Care for the exclusive supply of cannabis strains in Canada. "Through our relationship with Medropharm and Greenfields we not only gain access to certain in-demand high-CBD cannabis strains we will also benefit from their extensive research and innovation," INDIVA CEO Niel Marotta said.

Invictus *MD STRATEGIES CORP- (IVITF) 0.74*

Invictus hosts a platform for cannabis, located in Vancouver, the company wants to capitalize on the upcoming cannabis legalization process the federal government is set to take.

Invictus announced an agreement with Canopy Growth to allow the sale of the product from AB Labs, which was partly acquired by Invictus on the Tweed Main Street's online store. Invictus announced it had been included on the Horizons Marijuana Life Sciences Index ETF.

Kalytera Therapeutics *(HALTF) 0.044 (CALI*

Next on our stock list for cannabis investment is Kaltera. This clinical-stage pharmaceutical is working on developing the latest in therapies available through the use of cannabis. Kalytera is developing a new class of proprietary CBD therapeutics.

At the end of May, Kalytera announced its first quarter 2017 financial results, highlighting that the Canadian cannabis stock was spending $404,000 on research and development. In September the company received approval from the Institutional Review Board at one of two clinical sites in Israel to commence a Phase 2 study to evaluate cannabidiol (CBD) for the prevention of GvHD.

Khiron Life Sciences (KHIRNF) (2.30)

Khiron is a cannabis producer in Colombia raising capital in Canada through the TSX Venture Exchange. CEO Alvaro Torres told INN he wants to expand the strategy currently employed in Colombia for other Latin American markets such as Mexico.

Torres said as the Canadian market continues to grow with oversaturation investors will look to new opportunities like Colombia in the case of Khiron, with a patient population higher than the one in Canada.

Namaste Technologies (NXTTF) (0.81)

Namaste is a company offering consumers an entirely new platform where they can access and purchase vaporizer products from official manufacturers, and if allowed by the country medical cannabis. In Canada, the company has signed deals with licensed producers (LPs) to offer their products in the NamasteMD app. Through the mobile application, patients can obtain a prescription for medical marijuana.

Sean Dollinger, president, and CEO of Namaste told INN the company plans to launch a smartwatch app that will be able to collect data from the users after consuming cannabis products.

National Access Cannabis (NACNF) 0.48

This Canadian cannabis stock earned one of the coveted retail licenses for the province of Manitoba, which helped boost its share price so far in 2018. National Access Cannabis announced it was planning to strengthen its relationship with a few very different cannabis companies: CannaRoyalty, Cannabis Wheaton Income, and Tilray.

The license was a win for the company's decision to partner with the Nisichawayasihk Cree Nation of Manitoba to establish a retail recreational cannabis store in Thompson, Manitoba.

NATURALLY SPLENDID

Naturally Splendid has a slightly different focus than some of the other companies here on the Canadian cannabis stocks list. Rather than being involved in the medical marijuana space, the company offers investors exposure to the hemp-based healthy foods, omega, and cannabinoid markets.

The company announced it started shipping their NATERA(R) brand of products to an Australian distributor, opening the doors to a new cannabis market.

Newstrike Resources (TSXV:HIP)

Through its subsidiary, Up Cannabis, Newstrike

plans on developing various cannabis brands which would address medical client needs and as full legalization rolls into the country, recreational consumers as well. This licensed producer inked a deal with the Canadian band The Tragically Hip to contribute creatively to the company's efforts.

Shareholders of the Canadian cannabis stock voted in favor of being acquired by CanniMed Therapeutics (TSX:CMED) in January 2018, only for CanniMed to then cut a deal with Aurora Cannabis (TSX:ACB) and drop the potential acquisition of Newstrike.

OrganiGram Holdings *(OGRMF) (5.72)*

As its name suggests, OrganiGram specializes in producing organically grown medical marijuana. The company is licensed under the ACMPR and has a production facility located in Moncton, New Brunswick.

The Canadian cannabis stock has been actively involved with the business plan for the province of New Brunswick, it's home location. The company also announced a support agreement with le Collège Communautaire du Nouveau-Brunswick (CCNB) and the New Brunswick Department of Post-Secondary Education, Training and Labour "to support the delivery of the first commercial cannabis cultivation technician program in Canada."

Radient Technologies (RDDTF) (0.71)

Radient is an extraction technology company that has dabbled in the cannabis sector thanks to a partnership with licensed producer Aurora Cannabis. The partnership was unveiled this year and since then the two companies have provided an update on the status of their collaboration.

A press release from Aurora revealed the intention behind this partnership was to achieve a superior standardized cannabinoid extract.

"The potential to substantially increase our extracts production capacity while maintaining terpene profiles would further differentiate our Company, and we are excited to be exploring this opportunity further in the coming weeks," said Aurora's CEO Terry Booth in the same release.

Scythian Biosciences

Scythian is a research and development company with a patent application for the use of cannabinoids for the treatment of brain trauma injuries. This Canadian cannabis stock received a hefty investment from Aphria (TSX: APH), which acted as a leader of a private placement deal.

Tetra Bio-Pharma (TBPMF) 0.59

This Canadian cannabis stock operates in the drug discovery and development aspect of cannabis, more specifically cannabinoid-based drugs. Most recently the company obtained approval from Health Canadafor their phase 2 cannabis oil trial.

"We currently have a strong pipeline of five cannabinoid-based products, all launched last year and using different delivery systems, in various stages towards Health Canada and FDA approval," Bernard Fortier, CEO of Tetra Bio-Pharma's said.

The Supreme Cannabis Company (SPRWF) (1.41)

Supreme is next on our Canadian cannabis stocks list. Located in Kincardine, Ontario, the company's federally approved medical marijuana company, 7ACRES, cultivates medical marijuana on a greenhouse cost base. Along with 24 other companies, Supreme received its federal license.

In October the company announced its partner 7ACRES obtained Health Canada approvals in order to start cultivation at the recently completed 30,000 square feet flowering rooms at their hybrid facility.

WeedMD (WDDMF) (1.34)

Another officially licensed producer in Canada, WeedMD is focused on the growth of medical cannabis and sells its product directly to customers through their website. In May the company announced they received a sale license, which expands their business to include the sale of 1,200kg dried medicinal product per year.

Earlier this year the company joined the TSXV. The Canadian cannabis stock is looking to perform an expansion with a 220,000 square feet facility as it prepares for the recreational market to open in Canada. On June 28, it was announced that the company had entered a strategic partnership with Aurora Cannabis. Prior to that, WeedMD announced that it had secured a license from Health Canada to produce cannabis oils.

CANNABIS INVESTMENT: STOCKS ON THE CSE

The Canadian Securities Exchange (CSE) offers investors with a variety of cannabis-related companies seeking to increase their business activities. The CSE offers Canadian companies an option to seek business possibilities in the US, as long as it manages to disclose all its risks properly to shareholders. Let's take a look at some of the Canadian cannabis stocks listed there.

Abattis Bioceuticals (ATTBF) (0.049)

Abattis Bioceuticals is a vertically integrated biotechnology company focused on natural health products, including cannabis. The company develops natural health products and conducts research and development for the pharmaceutical, nutraceutical, bioceutical and cosmetic markets.

This year the Canadian cannabis stock has expanded their work in novel cannabis products with a partnership to develop a hemp-infused, cannabinoid-rich, THC-free craft beer alongside Vancouver-based craft brewery Faculty Brewing.

Alliance Growers (ALG WF) (0.070)

In its attempt to scale up on the cannabis market from a regional, national and international scope, ACG has moved to develop a Cannabis Botany Centre with Botanical Research In Motion International to jointly develop and operate multiple cannabis-focused Botany centers in Canada.

The Canadian cannabis stock provided an update to shareholders on their acquisition of

Biocannatech, a late-stage licensed producer applicant under Health Canada's access to cannabis for medical purposes regulations (ACMPR) in Quebec.

Beleave (BLEVF) (0.085)

Next on our stock list for cannabis investment is Beleave, a biotech company with a focus on becoming a licensed producer of medical-grade cannabis under the ACMPR. Its wholly-owned subsidiary, First Access, applied for a pre-license inspection in March 2017.

On January 31 the company announced it received a notification from Health Canada about its pre-sale inspection, which is now scheduled for February 8. If approved the Canadian cannabis stock will obtain a cannabis sales license.

Cannabix Technologies. (BLOZF) (1.27)

On the technology side of things, Cannabix Technologies is developing a breathalyzer that detects THC for use by law enforcement. The company announced its inclusion in the CSE25 Index in November 2017.

Most recently the company provided an update to shareholders of the development for their marijuana breathalyzer. "With completion of the modular Beta 3.0 prototype, Cannabix has achieved several key developmental milestones allowing this technology to be directly tested against the accepted laboratory standard of mass spectrometry," Chief Scientific Officer, Dr. Raj Attariwala said.

Canntab Therapeutics. (TLFTF) 0.68

Canntab is offering investors a different type of play into the cannabis market. The company develops cannabis oral dosage formulations thanks to exclusive technology working in the medical cannabis space.

This company officially launched its public stock on the CSE on April 20. "Canntab was able to take this step on only the second anniversary from its date of incorporation, and we intend to continue taking steps like these to enhance shareholder value, increase liquidity and execute on our strategic vision," Jeff Renwick, CEO and a director of Canntab said.

CannaRoyalty. (ORHOF) (7.10)

CannaRoyalty puts together its platform of holdings through royalty agreements, equity interests, convertible debt and licensing agreements across Canada and the US. The Canadian cannabis stock seeks to make investments in cannabis companies for the US market, with a direct focus on California, Nevada, and Florida.

After US Attorney General Jeff Sessions rescinded the Cole Memo, the company issued a statement reassuring shareholders of its position in the American market.

"The evidence from legal states demonstrates that legalizing and regulating cannabis consumption works," Marc Lusting, CEO of CannaRoyalty said. "It is our belief that this Memorandum has more to do with the DOJ's desire to ensure its ability to continue to enforce federal law without specific enforcement priorities regarding cannabis, than it does to disrupting ongoing state-legal cannabis activity."

CROP Infrastructure. (CRXPF)

CROP works with cannabis companies to offer capital for the acquisition of land real estate, branding and infrastructure for operations in the cannabis investment space.

This year the company has obtained 30 percent interest in facilities located in California and Washington State. "CROP continues to aggressively pursue new opportunities to expand its portfolio of tenant growers and infrastructure assets in strategic licensed jurisdictions," CROP director Alex Horsley said.

Friday Night Inc.

Friday Night is a cannabis producer based in the state of Nevada, one of the states to most recently legalized the recreational use of cannabis.

The company raised $7.5 million in order to fully capitalize on the high demand of the market in Las Vegas. On June 15, the company began trading on the CSE. Thanks to the boom of the Nevada market, the company is hoping to capitalize on the millions of tourists visiting Las Vegas.

The Canadian cannabis stock announced its intentions to expand its presence into one of the biggest cannabis market available, California.

FinCanna Capital (CSE:CALI)

Next on our stock list for cannabis investment is FinCanna, a royalty company for the licensed medical cannabis industry, with a focus on the California market. The company started trading on December 29, 2017.

Their lead investment is for Cultivation Technologies, which is planning the development of a production facility in Coachella, California.

FSD Pharma.

FSD is a Canadian cannabis company working on the development of an indoor hydroponic cultivation and processing facility, managed by its LP subsidiary FV Pharma. The company started trading on the CSE on May 29.

The facility the company is employing for its growth is a former KRAFT food manufacturing space in Cobourg, Ontario with a 620,000 square feet indoor facility. FSD counts with the support of

Auxly Cannabis through a joint-venture agreement. Based on the conditions of the deal Auxly will receive 49.9 percent of the cannabis produced in the facility. "It is anticipated that at full capacity this will result in FV receiving approximately 200,000,000 grams of dried cannabis flower per annum," FSD wrote in a statement.

Future Farm Technologies.

The company works on the development of agriculture technologies for the growth of plants. With the boom of the cannabis industry, Future Farm has expanded their business into marijuana, now representing one of their top 4 business priorities.

Through its subsidiaries, the Canadian cannabis stock has interests in farming projects in California related to the extraction of THC and CBD strains.

Global Cannabis Application.

Global Cannabis runs a mobile application business related to the cannabis industry. Their products include Citizen Green, Foro, Opinit and Truth.

The Canadian cannabis stock plans to roll out the launch of their cannabis lifestyle apps CannaLife and CannaMed. The company announced it will launch Citizen Green's CannaMed and CannaLife apps.

GLOBAL HEMP GROUP

Canadian cannabis stock Global Hemp focuses on the acquisition or joint venturing with companies all over the hemp and cannabis sector. The companies in their network include "suppliers of high quality sustainable raw materials and finished products derived from the hemp plant."

Global Hemp's latest joint venture is with Marijuana Company of America (OTC:MCOA) in which the two companies will work on the development of their New Brunswick hemp project.

Golden Leaf Holdings. (GLDFF) (0.0912)

Listed in Canada but located in Oregon, Golden

Leaf Holdings is focused on producing high-quality cannabis oils. Currently, the company's portfolio of brands is to meet the needs of patients, consumer and strategic partners.

The company gained licenses to sell its products in Las Vegas and other areas in the state of Nevada, a market that has expanded in 2017 with incredibly high demand, following the legalization of cannabis.

High Hampton Holdings. (HHPHF) (0.262)

Next on our stock list for cannabis investment is High Hampton, a cannabis operator focused on the Californian market. Through its subsidiary, CoachellaGro the company is expanding their reach in the state. As the company awaits for a Conditional Use Permit (CUP) for a 10.8-acre CoachellaGro facility located within the Coachella cultivation zone, in January it announced a strategic planning phase.

During the Lift Cannabis Expo in Vancouver this year, CEO David Argudo gave INN an update on the obstacles facing the California cannabis market. On the topic of risk potential for CSE-listed cannabis operators in the US, the company gave an update to shareholders after Canadian Securities Administrators issued a notice asking companies in this space for a risk disclosure update.

By further clarifying what is expected of an issuer, the CSA offers valuable guidance on disclosure necessities and further reiterates its commitment to follow this disclosure-based approach," Argudo said in the statement.

HIKU Brands Company.

Hiku is a Canadian cannabis stock whose company is focused on the lifestyle brand aspect of the industry. The company was created by the same team behind the popular Saxx Underwear.

Previously known as DOJA, the company completed a partnership with Tokyo Smoke to morph its public offering into HIKU. DOJA and all it's LP product are now a subsidiary of the new enterprise.

iAnthus. 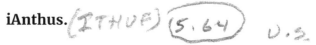 (ITHUF) (5.64) U.S.

This Canadian cannabis stock offers financing options to other cannabis cultivators, processors, and dispensaries in the US. The company has deals with licensed producers in four states: Colorado, Massachusetts, New Mexico and Vermont. By guiding these many companies iAnthus has a solid grasp on the cannabis sector in America.

iAnthus currently has almost 20 million invested in five cannabis operations since the start of 2016. "We look forward to making additional investments in greenfield states as well as acquiring assets that have strong track records of revenue growth and cash flow generation," Julius Kalcevich, CFO of iAnthus, said in a statement.

The Canadian cannabis stock made a push for the Florida market by buying the assets of GrowHealthy Holdings a local Florida company.

InMed Pharmaceuticals. (IMLFF) (0.38)

InMed is developing therapies for patients through the research of cannabinoids in combination with drug delivery systems. The company has a dermatology product with clinical trials planned all throughout 2020. VANCOUVER, CAN

The Canadian cannabis stock recently shared some results from its co-sponsored study with the University of British Columbia. "The InMed-UBC study is the first ever to report hydrogel-mediated cannabinoid nanoparticle delivery to the eye, resulting in enhanced drug uptake via the cornea and lens," InMed said.

Isodiol International. (ISOLF) (1.013)

Through its own online store, Isodiol offers a variety of cannabidiol (CBD) products like oils,

VANCOUVER, CAN

sprays, and patches. The company has developed proprietary ISO 9001 and GMP-certified cannabinoid production and purification methods to formulate high-quality CBD products.

Isodiol is one of the first Canadian companies to express an interest in entering the Mexican market, following medical legalization in the country. Isodiol announced in early July that it had received approval from the Brazilian Health Regulatory Agency for its pharmaceutical grade Cannabidiol product, Isoderm.

Lexaria Bioscience (LXRP) (1.03)

Lexaria is food biosciences company that has the technology for improved delivery of bioactive compounds. In particular, the Canadian cannabis stock offers a variety of hemp oil products to its consumers and also has some novel food offerings like a black tea infused with hemp oil.

KELOWNA, CAN

Lexaria has filed patents in the US to protect their lipid-based delivery mechanisms. On October 31, the company announced it received a US patent for the use of its "technology as a delivery platform for all cannabinoids including THC; fat-soluble vitamins; non-steroidal anti-inflammatory pain medications; and nicotine."

Lineage Grow Company.

Lineage is a company focused on holding a lineup of licensed producer assets across the US and Canada. The company currently is seeking assets in Oregon, California, Maryland and Pennsylvania.

In June the company announced an agreement to acquire Agris Farms, a premium quality craft cannabis cultivation company in Northern California.

Koios Beverage *CORP — (KBEVF) 0.25*

Koios is a company working on the development of a beverage for brain health purposes. In May the

VANCOUVER, CAN.

company announced the start of official testing into patients using the Koios products by the NeuraPerformance/Neuroptimize BrainCente. These centers will soon start offering the beverages in its locations.

"Not only will this clinical trial further substantiate our product formulation, but the data collected will pave the way to creating better technologies within our portfolio," Chris Miller, CEO of Koios said.

Lotus Ventures. *(LTTSF) (0.183)*

Lotus is a medical marijuana company planning to build a 28,000 square foot facility. Lotus is awaiting a confirmation letter from Health Canada regarding their federal license.

Recently the Canadian cannabis stock announced it had signed a deal with Cannabis Wheaton (TSXV:CBW) for $5 million worth of common shares.

Liberty Health Sciences. (LHSIF)

(handwritten: Toronto .66 / LHSIF 0.81)

Liberty Health is a company focused on cannabis opportunities in the US. They are partnered with Aphria (TSX:APH; OTCQB:APHQF) Currently, Liberty Health is focused on the market available in Florida, including a variety of deals to provide cannabis products to that state.

Liberty Leaf. (LIBFF)

(handwritten: 0.11 / 0.086 / VANCOUVER CANADA)

Liberty Leaf Holdings is focused on the business of acquiring partnership interests in up-and-coming and established companies in the medicinal and recreational cannabis investment space. On October 27, the Canadian cannabis stock announced it received an aggregate $763,500 from the exercise of share purchase warrants.

Marapharm Ventures. (LIHTF)

(handwritten: Liht Cannabis Corp .645 / .15 / LIHTF 0.22)

Next on our stock list for cannabis investment is Marapharm Ventures. The company has two operations in British Columbia. The company's

(handwritten: Kelowna, Canada)

initial facility–a proposed 22,000 square feet area –will be on an 11-acre site in Kelowna.

Marapharm has also purchased land in Las Vegas for the purpose of building a facility that will host three medical marijuana licenses. What's more, the company also has the opportunity in Washington to lease a facility to a tier 3 license holder.

WAYLAND GROUP Corp. (MRRCF)

Maricann. 0.43 .43 BURlington, CANADA

Maricann is relatively new to the Canadian cannabis stocks, having joined the CSE under the symbol MARI on April 24th. Maricann expects to be finished with the construction of their Langton facility in 2017, which will up their production square footage from 44,000 to 217,500.

The company gave shareholders an update on its recent financing options, including increasing "the size of the Offering from up to $20,000,000 aggregate principal amount of Convertible

Debenture Units to up to $26,000,000 (or up to $31,000,000, factoring in the full exercise of the Agents' Option (as defined below))."

Matica Enterprises. (MQPXF)

[handwritten: Toronto, CAN] [handwritten: 0.097] [handwritten: 0.080]

Matica is involved in the acquisition of 70 percent of a late stage ACMPR applicant and builds a 10,000 square foot facility in Quebec.

This facility received its official inspection by the management team of Matica, with CEO Boris Zieger saying their facility is on schedule and should be done by November of 2017.

MedMen Enterprises. (MMNFF)

[handwritten: Culver City, CA] [handwritten: 3.00] [handwritten: 3.29]

MedMen is a cannabis dispensary operator focused on the US market. The company owns dispensaries in key states like California and Nevada and has been able to hold onto a popularity to its branding and promotion.

MedMen signed onto a partnership with LP Cronos Group for a joint venture and the creation of MedMen Canada, this new entity will oversee the creation of cannabis dispensaries in Canada modeled similarly to the popular MedMen stores in the US.

MPX Bioceutical Corporation (CSE:BCC)

Through its subsidiaries and investments in several states in the US, MPX Bioceutical Corporation is involved in the American cannabis market. Formerly known as Canadian Bioceutical Corporation, the company officially changed its name in November.

The company applied for a Canadian licensed producer (LP) status, but due to a rocky unresponsive process decided to mobilize its investments in the US. On May 22, 2017, the company officially began trading on the OTCQB Market.

(BCCEF) 0.0242?

MYM Nutraceuticals (CSE:MYM) *(MYMMF) (1.48)*

VANCOUVER, CANADA

Our next Canadian cannabis stocks company is MYM Nutraceuticals, another biopharmaceutical company, and distributor of medical marijuana. It has applied to Health Canada for a production license under MMPR and considers itself well prepared for distribution of medical marijuana, and a growing facility property.

The company has performed a strategy seeking the Australian market, on November 14 the company announced it had completed multiple patent filings with the Office of Drug Control.

NanoSphere. *(NSHSF) (0.35) (.26) Colorado*

NanoSphere is a biotech company working on novel delivery methods. Their relation to the cannabis industry comes in the form of technology. Most recently the Canadian cannabis stock announced a deal with a private-label manufacturer of pharmaceutical goods based in California.

"This new venture not only opens up a huge market, but is a fantastic opportunity to increase our visibility and reputation in the legal cannabis investment space, and represents a significant stepping stone to reaching even more new patients and consumers with our lauded transdermal delivery system," Robert Sutton, Chairman and CEO at NanoSphere said.

Nutritional High.

Nutritional High is a Canadian cannabis stock focused on cannabis-infused edible products and oil extracts for both the medical and recreational market. On October 8, the company announced it was entering into a novel cannabis market: beverages. The company "entered into an agreement with Xanthic Biopharma to manufacture and distribute their innovative cannabis-infused powdered drinks and other products in Colorado.

Phivida Holdings. (PHVAF) 0.38 .51 VANCOUVER, CANADA

Next on our stock list for cannabis investment is Phivida. The company works on CBD infused foods and beverages and clinical CBD products. Most recently the company announced an agreement with Namaste Technologies (CSE:N; OTCMKTS:NXTTF) to distribute their products in Germany and Australia.

"This Agreement represents a pilot project between both companies whereby Namaste will distribute Phivida's proprietary CBD beverages and infused products within the designated territories," the companies announced on their joint statement.

PUF Ventures. (PUFXF) 0.22 4/3 VANCOUVER CANADA

PUF Ventures has a diversified portfolio of assets in the Canadian marijuana sector. It owns a passive, non-controlling interest in AAA Heidelberg, which is focused on using all-natural nutrients to grow healthy, pest-free plants.

AAA Heidelberg has had an MMPR application pending with Health Canada since 2013. Other ventures the company has invested in include 1313 Cigs, VapeTronix, and Weed Beacon. In late January, the Canadian cannabis stock announced it had recommenced its development of the WeedBacon platform.

BURNABY, BC

Quadron Capital Corporation. (QCC) 0.165

Quadron works to help licensed producers in Canada with "complex needs and requirements" through equipment, products, and services. The company also offers dispensing devices and consumption products. The company has two subsidiaries in Soma Labs Scientific, Greenmantle, and Cybernetic Control Systems.

During its most recent financial disclosure, the Canadian cannabis stock announced an increase in revenue to $516,211 during their first quarter.

RISE Life Science. _Corp. (MCUIF) (0.17)_ _TORONTO, CAN._

RISE Life Science is a company developing cannabis consumer products for both medical and adult-use markets. The company plans to establish a potential capacity in 2019 to market all of its CBD products throughout the US, Canadian and European markets.

In June the company provided shareholders with a corporate update to project the entry of sexual health cannabis products this year. "RISE products are expected to be available in California retail locations by the end of July and will be offered through dispensaries initially, followed by health food retailers and natural wellness boutiques," the company indicated.

TerrAscend. _(TRSSF) (6.12)_ _Mississauga CANADA_

Another fairly new member of the Canadian cannabis stocks is TerrAscend, who went public in May 2017 when it entered the Canadian Securities Exchange. The company's subsidiary, Solace

Health, is in the process of applying for an official licensing designation from Health Canada. Solace is host to a 67,000 square feet production facility

The company's other subsidiary Terra Health Network is a research-based cannabinoid medical group, which wants to improve the medical cannabis solutions available for patients with chronic pain and debilitating illnesses.

Kelowna, CANADA

THC Biomed. *(THC BF) 0.34*

Next on our stock list for cannabis investment is THC Biomed, who has been granted permission to conduct research and development for scientific purposes with medicinal marijuana. The company provides scientific and biotechnical services to current and potential licensed producers. In May 2016, Health Canada granted TCH BioMed a license to produce fresh marijuana, cannabis oil, and cannabis resin.

Tinley Beverage (TNYBF) (0.5D) *TORONTO, CANADA*

Tinley Beverage is the producer of Hemplify, a drinkable vitality supplement containing hemp extract made from the stalk of industrial hemp. The vegan, sugar-free drink is a source of electrolytes, vitamins and Omega 3 fatty acids. The company reported receiving its first orders for Hemplify products on March.

True Leaf Medicine. (TRLFF) (0.32) *VERNON, CANADA*

Canada-based True Leaf is slightly different than the afore-mentioned Canadian cannabis stocks; the company is focused on the production of hemp-based functional dog chews. In August 2016, the company secured the first order for its True Hemp pet products with Pets Corner, the second largest pet store chain in the United Kingdom. The store will sell the product in all of its 174 stores. The sale also means that True Hemp is now generating revenue on two continents – North America and Europe. "We're on our way to becoming a truly global brand," said CEO Darcy Bomford.

Kelowna, Canada

Valens GroWorks. (VGWCF) (1.99)

Located in British Columbia's Okanagan Valley, our next Canadian cannabis stocks is Valens GroWorks, a "rapidly emerging" with a focus on cannabis cultivation and research. In November the company announced it had increased a private placement offer in order to advance the operational capability of its Kelowna Facility.

Veritas Pharma. (VDRSF) (0.092) Delta Canada

Veritas is working on fully understanding the medical capabilities of marijuana, the company's mission is to find the most effective strains that target a specific disease condition. Veritas is using a specifically designed approach to their research where they chemically and pharmacologically profile the plant. As a last check, they completed a clinical study of each cultivar.

Vinergy Resources.

Vinergy is an oil and gas company, that acquired MJ BioPharma, a cannabis technology company focused on manufacturing breath strips, time release capsules, extract oils, food products, and infused juices, teas, coffee and extract drinks and pharmaceutical grade delivery systems.

The pair announced in February the had developed an oral cannabinoid complex delivery strips and controlled time release capsule technology. "We think time release capsules are extremely important as they help bridge the gap in terms of familiarity with many patients who want to switch from synthetic drugs to a natural product as a way to reduce side effects and drug," said Mr. Kent Deuters, CEO of MJ Biopharma.

Vodis Pharmaceuticals.

Next on our stock list for cannabis investment is Vodis. The firm has medical and recreational marijuana business operations in both Canada and the United States. With facilities in BC and Washington State, Vodis is actively seeking expansion opportunities in other countries and US states.

In March, the company announced it, together with Our Church International, signed a 15-year licensing and marketing agreement. Later that month, Vodis announced construction had begun on its Bellingham cannabis facility. Following that, the Canadian cannabis stock announced its USA-branded product had begun selling in Washington State. On June 20, Vodis announced a $5 million private placement financing.

VANCOUVER, CANADA

Wildflower Brands. (WLDFF) (0.50)

Working exclusively in Washington State, Wildflower Marijuana lists in Canada, with a focus on developing and designing products in the cannabis sector.

On June 27, Wildflower announced that its products would soon be coming to Amazon.com—which shouldn't come as a surprise. Earlier in June, the company announced a brand expansion into the American market.

(handwritten: 4.338)

Xanthic Biopharma. *(handwritten: (GGBYF) GREEN GRD... BRANDS INC)*

Last but not least on our stock list for cannabis investment is Xanthic. It is a company working with strategic partners to deliver a higher quality of cannabinoid solubility, improved bioavailability, accurate micro-dosing and greater consistency versus competitive infused products, thanks to a patent-pending process.

In May a strategic partner of the company, Avitas CBD Water, rebranded into Xanthic Beverages. "With a business model focused on licensing our water-soluble technology and brand name to qualified producers, being able to demonstrate initial success on the West Coast of the US with

Xanthic CBD Water will be extremely valuable," Tim Moore, CEO of Xanthic said.

(MGWFF) 0.17

Maple Leaf Green World (NEO: MGW) Calgary, CANADA

Maple Leaf is a company with interests in both the Canadian and US cannabis markets. The company's facility in Telkwa, B.C. is in the process of applying for federal license to grow medical marijuana under the Access to Cannabis for Medical Purposes Regulations (ACMPR). In the US the company holds a medical cultivation license in Nevada and is seeking a recreational one as well.

In 2018 Maple Leaf elected to drop the TSXV Exchange, in which it previously traded for the fairly new Aequitas NEO Exchange, a first of its kind move in the cannabis space.

Do you want to venture into the cannabis investment space? Why or why not?

Did we miss a company that you think should be included on the Canadian cannabis stocks list? Let us know in the comments!

This article has been updated since its original publication in 2016, with the most recent update done by Bryan Mc Govern.

California Cannabis Investing: Understanding 'Ownership' and 'Financial Interests

Passage of California's Medicinal and Adult-Use Cannabis Regulation and Safety Act ("MAUCRSA") has opened the doors to institutional investing in California cannabis companies. California's lack of a residency requirement for investors and its relatively limited investor disclosure and background requirements have made it popular for institutional investors looking to invest in cannabis.

There are two main types of California cannabis applicants: owners and financial interest holders. To be legally considered an "owner" under California's cannabis regulations, one does not actually need equity in the applicant's cannabis business. "Owner" means any of the following:

A person with an aggregate ownership interest of 20 percent or more in the person applying for a license or a licensee, unless the interest is solely a security, lien, encumbrance;

The chief executive officer of a nonprofit or other entity;

A member of the board of directors of a nonprofit; and

Any individual who will be participating in the direction, control, or management of the person applying for a license.

An individual who directs, controls, or manages the business includes any of the following: a partner of a commercial cannabis business that is organized as a partnership; a member of a limited liability company of a commercial cannabis business that is organized as a limited liability company; and an officer or director of a commercial cannabis business that is organized as a corporation.

AL TALK NETWORK

Even if someone is not an "owner," that person or company may still be deemed a financial interest holder ("FIH"). "Financial interest" means "an investment into a commercial cannabis business, a loan provided to a commercial cannabis business, or any other 'equity interest' in a commercial cannabis business." California cannabis regulators consider the term "equity interest" to include less than a 20 percent ownership in the cannabis applicant and pretty much any profit-sharing arrangement or entitlement to profits from cannabis licensees including IP licensing royalties and percentage rent arrangements. The following are not considered FIHs: banks and financial institutions; diversified mutual funds, blind trusts, or similar instruments; holders of security interests, liens, or encumbrances on property that will be used by the commercial cannabis business; and individuals holding less than 5 percent of the total shares in a publicly traded company.

California requires FIHs be disclosed to and vetted by the state upon application for annual cannabis licenses and the license applicants must provide a list of all financing it receives. Specifically, the license application mandates applicants include the name, birthdate, and government-issued identification type and number (i.e., driver's license) for any individual with a financial interest in a commercial cannabis business. FIHs are not required to submit to criminal background checks, but they will still undergo some vetting by state regulators.

Even with these new rules, most institutional investment in the cannabis space is still concentrated in "ancillary services" — those services that support cannabis businesses but do not "touch the plant." Examples include turnkey real estate, equipment and materials leasing and sales, IP licensing, consulting services, and tech platforms. Many institutional investors still want to stay one or two steps removed from touch-the-plant cannabis businesses and do not like the idea of being listed in a state database as being an owner or FIH. However, given California's wide-reaching definition of owner and FIH, even these companies and their investors can be deemed by the state to have this direct cannabis business interest. To avoid being considered owners or FIHs in California, ancillary service providers will need to avoid directly providing financing, using profit-sharing or similar performance-based payment schemes with cannabis businesses, and they will also need to avoid managing, directing, or controlling the licensed entity.

MARIJUANA STOCKS AND OTHER WAYS TO INVEST IN CANNABIS

There are many people who are making money from legal cannabis. MMJ has created jobs that didn't exist just a few years ago. Some of these opportunities are limited to people living in states with relaxed pot laws. Others are available to all of us.

How can investors and entrepreneurs take advantage of this trend? Let's look at 9 market and business opportunities available for those who choose to enter the legitimate marijuana market, from investing in marijuana stocks to other opportunities.

Grower

It all starts with the seeds and plants. Growing marijuana is a science. Individuals can start with just few plants as allowed by state law. The larger organizations employ master growers, hydroponics farmers, and botanists. Think of this like a professional agriculture operation – if legalization occurs, mainstream farmers may switch to this crop as well.

In fact, the University of Mississippi has restarted it's "legal" growing operation to fund studies for various government departments all over the United States. This is a good sign for other marijuana growers.

Dispensary

The dispensaries take on lots of risk. They are the pharmacies that sell medical marijuana. However, they have doors to kick down, and the Federal government does it regularly. But that hasn't stopped them from spreading all over cities in California, Arizona, Colorado, and other states.

Delivery Service

Delivery drivers will bring cannabis right to your door. A great opportunity for those looking to get into the weed business with minimal investment.

If you've been following the news later, Uber, Google, Amazon, and more are getting into the specialty delivery space. You can even do side hustles as a delivery driver with companies like Post Mates. Adding in marijuana will only grow this area.

Contractor

Electricians, construction crews, and irrigation experts are all needed to build large-scale grow operations. Many cities in areas where medical marijuana is legal already have hydroponic shops that have experts in these areas.

In fact, several investment firms have focused specifically on this area, including GreenGro Technologies. Just building the equipment and spaces required in the industry can be lucrative.

Trimmer & Bud Tender

Trimmers clean up the buds and make them pretty before sale. This seemingly boring job can pay very well. Bud tenders work at dispensaries, ringing up customers and providing them with advice on different strains. Think of it as the sommelier of marijuana.

Device Maker

A large sub-market. There are a variety of device makers making and selling grinders, glass smoking devices, smoking paraphernalia etc. Vaporizers are a very popular area of this market. Many smoke shops are already selling a variety of devices for tobacco use that are used for marijuana.

In fact, Seattle company mCig Inc. is an herbal cigarette and vaporizer maker that has explicitly stated it's focusing on the marijuana market.

Online Entrepreneur

Weedmaps is a great example of how legal weed gave someone the chance to create an entirely new business. And that's just one example. Countless blogs, weed-themed stores, review sites, and other businesses make money for online entrepreneurs.

Venture Capitalist

As cannabis goes mainstream, the big money moves in. Forbes reports that venture capitalists are investing cash in the industry. Leafly is one example. The cannabis review and dispensary website is a venture capitalist backed MMJ business.

Stock Investor

Not everyone is cut out for the weed business. And not all of us have deep pockets like a venture capitalist. But you can still profit from cannabis. Investors can buy marijuana stocks.

Also, be careful because investing in marijuana stocks can get you fired in some cases.

Legal cannabis presents unique and interesting opportunities for investors and entrepreneurs. Once it is legalized on a federal level, it will become a major part of the US economy. There is money to be made in this emerging industry.

How to Invest in a Cannabis Stock

It's no secret that the cannabis sector is one of the hottest commodities currently out there, with companies rushing to be publicly listed to get in on the action.

Putting it simply, investor interest in cannabis – both sophisticated and those new to the market– is heating up, but before any investor makes the decision to enter this market, there are a number of key decisions that need to be made.

With that in mind, the goal of the Investing News Network (INN) is to educate investors and help make key decisions with respect to their portfolios. Here, INN asked some experts in the cannabis industry some of the most important questions every investor should ask to better understand how to invest in a cannabis stock.

How to invest in a cannabis stock: does the company have a license?

One of the most crucial–if not most crucial–components of any cannabis company is the type of license they may hold or a license they could be applying for in the future.

Following an arduous review process companies can qualify to obtain Licenced Producer status from Health Canada under the Access to Cannabis for Medical Purpose Regulations, this may give the company a visibility boost based on the fact that currently there are only 48 licensed producers in the country. The company may gain a recognition of solid business practice–at least according to the health agency.

The acquisition of a Health Canada officiated licensed producer status for a cannabis producer equals a boost in visibility and a certification of solid business practice–at least according to the health agency.

Sean Gercsak, an investment advisor with Canaccord Genuity Wealth Management who's had experience raising capital for companies in this sector, said licensed producers in Canada have seen impressive gains in their stocks over the last 24 months.

The knowledge of what type of license–if any at all–a company holds can paint a clearer picture of where the company is heading and if it's worth investing in.

Depending on the stage of the licensing process, generating revenue could be anywhere from days to months to years away.

How to invest in a cannabis stock: does the management team have experience?

Like any other industry, as an investor the need to have a solid awareness of a company's management team is crucial.

These are people you're entrusting your money to, and if you can't be confident about that then, by all means, don't invest.

The first thing an investor should find out about the people involved in the administration of the company is their experience in the market and their established relationship to the industry.

Two key indicators of an experienced management team include people who may have strong, large-scale greenhouse growing experience," or people with executive experience from the pharmaceutical world – preferably someone involved with the launch of a blockbuster drug of some kind.

Is management only here to make money, or do they have previous experience on the other side of the table where cannabis made a material impact on their symptoms?Together, these give a strong backing towards management's passion for the industry and building their company.

How to invest in a cannabis stock: what does its capital structure look like?

A quick review of any public company's financial sheets will provide a lot of information into the model of the company, such as warrants and options.

What's more recommended that investors find out how many shares management holds, if they have been buying or selling their own shares, and how much capital the founders first put into the company.

Brown added that investors should check if there are dilutive securities and what their exercise prices are as well as the prices and valuations previous financings were done at if a financing closed recently. He also said investors should know if the shares have a free-trading hold period, it's worthwhile knowing when that period ends.

Another important fact to know in terms of capital structure is if the company is currently facing any debt. This could prove important as the company continues working towards its goals.

Finally, investors might want to ask a company how much are its cash savings, and for how long will that keep the company afloat before they need to raise more capital?

What's more, Brown recommended that investors find out how many shares management holds, if they have been buying or selling their own shares, and how much capital the founders first put into the company.

Investors should check if there are dilutive securities and what their exercise prices are as well as the prices and valuations previous financings were done at if a financing closed recently. He also said investors should know if the shares have a free-trading hold period, it's worthwhile knowing when that period ends.

Another important fact to know in terms of capital structure is if the company is currently facing any debt. This could prove important as the company continues working towards its goals.

Finally, investors might want to ask a company how much are its cash savings, and for how long will that keep the company afloat before they need to raise more capital?

INVESTMENT OPPORTUNITIES

There are many different opportunities for investors within Canada's cannabis industry.

Licensed producers represent the largest and most pure-play option for investors since they enjoy exclusive rights to grow, harvest, and process marijuana into flowers, extracts, and edibles.

Ancillary markets, such as testing labs, infused-product makers, and security firms, are poised to capture a further $13.9 billion in annual revenue, according to Deloitte. While the revenue opportunity is larger, there are many more companies targeting these areas of the market compared to less than 50 licensed producers due to government restrictions. These companies offer the opportunity to diversify away from purely growing into ancillary industries.

Risk Factors to Consider

Cannabis has widely used for thousands of years, but since the 1940s, the drug has become illegal in many countries thanks to the U.S.-led War on Drugs. In a surprising twist, the U.S. has become among the first major countries to begin decriminalizing the drug on a state-by-state level. Despite these trends, the drug remains illegal in many countries and faces regulatory risks on a federal level in the United States.

Canada's cannabis industry may be well-established on a federal level, but there are still many risks that investors should consider. Companies operating in the space could face risks when it comes to exporting the drug, which could become an issue over time as the domestic market becomes saturated and export markets become a key growth driver. Many companies are also traded over-the-counter with somewhat limited trading volume in the U.S.

Canada may be best-known for its energy and precious metals industries, but the cannabis industry has emerged as its fastest-growing industry. In addition to 38 licensed producers, there are hundreds of other companies that produce ancillary products and services. Investors may want to consider these companies for their portfolios, although it's important to be cognizant of the risks associated with these companies and the wider industry.

CONCLUSION

Marijuana is one of the most abused drugs in the world. There is an ever-growing gap between the latest science about marijuana and the myths surrounding it. Some people think that since it is legal in some places, it must be safe. But your body doesn't know a legal drug from an illegal drug. It only knows the effect the drug creates once you have taken it.

Marijuana, when sold, is a mixture of dried out leaves, stems, flowers and seeds of the hemp plant. It is usually green, brown or gray in color.

Hashish is tan, brown or black resin that is dried and pressed into bars, sticks or balls. When smoked, both marijuana and hashish give off a distinctive, sweet odor.

There are over 400 chemicals in marijuana and hashish. The chemical that causes intoxication or the "high" in users is called THC (short for tetrahydrocannabinol). THC creates the mind-altering effects that classifies marijuana as a drug.

Plants, like animals, have traits that protect them in the wild. Plants can have colors or patterns that camouflage them from predators, or they can contain poisons or toxins that, when eaten, make animals sick or alter their mental capacity, putting them at risk in the wild. THC is the protective mechanism of the marijuana plant.

Intoxication literally means "to poison by taking a toxic substance into your body." Any substance that intoxicates causes changes in the body and the mind. It can create addiction or dependence, causing a person to want to take that drug even if it harms him or her.

You may have heard someone say that because marijuana is a plant, it's "natural" and so it's harmless. But it's not.

Marijuana can be smoked as a cigarette (joint), but may also be smoked in a dry pipe or a water pipe known as a "bong." It can also be mixed with food and eaten or brewed as tea.

With all that said, would a reasonable person invest in cannabis stocks for the long haul, the answer is a 100% "Heck Yes"!

Good Luck with your investing and God bless you.

If you found any value is this book can you please take a moment a leave a review on Amazon and tell us about your cannabis story.

Thank you again for your support!

PAYPAC

288-227-1161

456645

24787475R00075

Made in the USA
San Bernardino, CA
07 February 2019